ACHIEVING PEAK PERFORMANCE

The Blueprint For Bodybuilding Advancement

Ronald L Abrams

Table of Content

INTRODUCTION

Welcome to the realm of bodybuilding, where sculpting the physique becomes an art form, and achieving peak performance is the ultimate quest. In this dynamic arena, success is not merely measured in muscle mass but in the intricate balance of discipline, dedication, and strategic planning.

To embark on this journey is to enter a world where every repetition, every meal, and every ounce of effort contributes to the blueprint of your body's transformation. It's a pursuit that demands more than physical exertion; it requires mental fortitude, nutritional precision, and a relentless pursuit of excellence.

In this guide, we delve into the intricacies of achieving peak performance in bodybuilding. From understanding the science behind muscle growth to crafting personalized training regimens and optimizing nutrition, we unravel the secrets that propel athletes from average to exceptional.

But beyond the weights and protein shakes lies a deeper narrative—a story of resilience, perseverance, and the unwavering commitment to surpassing one's limitations. It's about embracing the journey as much as the destination, finding purpose in every rep, and channeling the relentless pursuit of progress into every aspect of life.

So, whether you're a seasoned competitor or a newcomer to the world of bodybuilding, join me as we explore the blueprints for advancement, uncovering the strategies, techniques, and mindset shifts that pave the way to realizing your full potential in the pursuit of peak performance.

Definitions

1. Accomplishment: Achievement can be defined as the successful completion or attainment of a goal, task, or objective, often requiring effort, skill, or perseverance.

- Achievement also encompasses the acknowledgment or recognition of one's efforts, abilities, or contributions, whether by oneself or by others.

- Personal Fulfillment: Beyond tangible outcomes, achievement can represent a sense of personal fulfillment, satisfaction, or growth resulting from overcoming challenges, reaching milestones, or realizing aspirations.

2. Summit/Peak of a Mountain: The highest point of a mountain, often used metaphorically to represent reaching the highest level or achievement in a particular domain.

- Maximum/Peak Performance: The highest level of performance or functioning that an individual or system can achieve, often implying optimal efficiency or effectiveness.

- Population/Peak of Activity: The highest level or point of activity, popularity, or usage reached by something, such as a product, trend, or phenomenon.

3. Blueprints can represent strategic plans or frameworks outlining the steps, goals, and resources needed to achieve a particular objective or vision, especially in business or organizational contexts.

Definitions of terms in bodybuilding

Here are some common terms in bodybuilding:

1. Rep (Repetition): One complete movement of an exercise, usually from the starting position to the end and back again.

2. Set: A group of consecutive repetitions of an exercise.

3. Superset: Performing two exercises back-to-back with no rest in between.

4. Compound Exercise: An exercise that targets multiple muscle groups simultaneously, such as squats or bench presses.

5. Isolation Exercise: An exercise that targets a specific muscle group, such as bicep curls or tricep extensions.

6. Bulk: A phase of training and dieting aimed at gaining muscle mass.

7. Cut: A phase of training and dieting aimed at reducing body fat while maintaining muscle mass.

8. Muscle Definition: The visibility of muscle shape and separation due to low body fat.

9. Rep Range: The number of repetitions performed per set, typically categorized as low (1-5 reps), moderate (6-12 reps), or high (12+ reps).

10. Failure: Reaching the point where you can no longer perform additional reps with proper form.

11. Hypertrophy: The increase in muscle size due to an increase in the size of individual muscle fibers.

12. Strength Training: Training focused on increasing maximal strength, often involving lower rep ranges and heavier weights.

13. Pump: The temporary increase in muscle size due to increased blood flow during exercise.

14. Macros (Macronutrients): The three main nutrients that provide energy: protein, carbohydrates, and fats.

15. Cutting Cycle: A period of time during which a bodybuilder reduces calorie intake to lose body fat while maintaining muscle mass.

16. Bulking Cycle: A period of time during which a bodybuilder increases calorie intake to gain muscle mass.

17. DOMS (Delayed Onset Muscle Soreness): The muscle soreness that occurs 24-72 hours after intense exercise.

18. Toning: A term often used to describe the process of reducing body fat and increasing muscle definition.

19. Body Fat Percentage: The proportion of fat to lean mass in the body, often measured using various methods like calipers or bioelectrical impedance analysis.

20. Peak: The state of maximum muscle fullness and vascularity achieved through specific training, diet, and hydration strategies, often before a competition.

** 1 **

SETTING GOALS: THE FOUNDATION OF SUCCESS

Setting goals is like charting a course for success. It provides direction, motivation, and a sense of purpose. When you set clear and achievable goals, you give yourself something to strive for, helping you stay focused and organized. Goals act as a roadmap, guiding your actions and decisions towards desired outcomes. They also provide a way to measure progress and celebrate achievements along the way, which boosts morale and keeps you moving forward. In essence, setting goals lays the groundwork for success by providing a clear path and keeping you accountable to your aspirations.

Setting goals is indeed the bedrock of achieving success. Here's a breakdown of why:

1. **Clarity**: Goals provide clarity about what you want to achieve, giving you a clear target to aim for.

2. **Motivation**: They fuel motivation by creating a sense of purpose and direction, helping you stay focused and committed to your objectives.

3. **Focus**: Goals help you prioritize tasks and activities, preventing distractions and ensuring that your efforts are aligned with your desired outcomes.

4. **Measurement**: They offer a way to measure progress and success, allowing you to track your achievements and make adjustments if necessary.

5. **Challenge**: Setting goals challenges you to push beyond your comfort zone, fostering personal and professional growth.

6. **Accountability**: By setting specific goals, you hold yourself accountable for taking action and achieving results.

7. **Decision Making**: Having clear goals simplifies decision-making processes, as you can evaluate choices based on whether they support your objectives.

Overall, setting goals provides a roadmap for success, guiding your actions and decisions towards realizing your aspirations.

HOW TO SET GOALS FOR SUCCESS

Setting goals for success involves several key steps:

1. **Define Your Objectives**: Clearly articulate what you want to achieve. Make sure your goals are specific, measurable, achievable, relevant, and time-bound (SMART).

2. **Identify Your Priorities**: Determine what matters most to you and prioritize your goals accordingly. Focus on the goals that will have the biggest impact on your success.

3. **Break Down Your Goals**: Divide your goals into smaller, manageable tasks or milestones. This makes them less overwhelming and easier to track progress.

4. **Create an Action Plan**: Develop a detailed plan outlining the steps you need to take to reach each goal. Include deadlines and checkpoints to stay on track.

5. **Stay Flexible**: Be open to adjusting your goals and action plan as needed. Circumstances may change, and it's important to adapt accordingly.

6. **Stay Motivated**: Find ways to stay inspired and motivated, whether it's through visualizing your success, seeking support from others, or celebrating small victories along the way.

7. **Monitor Your Progress**: Regularly review your goals and track your progress. This allows you to identify any areas where you may need to make adjustments or put in extra effort.

8. **Stay Persistent**: Success often requires perseverance and resilience. Stay committed to your goals, even when faced with challenges or setbacks.

By following these steps, you can set yourself up for success and increase your chances of achieving your goals.

FACTORS THAT CAN HINDER YOU FROM ACHIEVING YOUR GOALS

Here are several factors that can hinder you from achieving your goals:

1. **Lack of clarity**: Unclear goals make it difficult to determine the necessary steps for achievement.

2. **Procrastination**: Delaying tasks or actions needed to progress towards your goals can impede success.

3. **Fear of failure**: Being afraid to fail may prevent you from taking risks or trying new approaches.

4. **Distractions**: Focusing on non-essential activities instead of prioritizing tasks relevant to your goals can slow progress.

5. **Negative mindset**: Pessimism or self-doubt can undermine motivation and confidence, making it harder to persevere.

6. **Lack of planning**: Failing to create a structured plan with actionable steps can lead to aimless efforts and wasted time.

7. **Inconsistency**: Not maintaining consistent effort and dedication towards your goals can result in slow or stagnant progress.

8. **Lack of resources**: Insufficient access to necessary tools, knowledge, or support can hinder your ability to achieve your goals effectively.

9. **Overcommitment**: Spreading yourself too thin by pursuing too many goals simultaneously can lead to burnout and reduced effectiveness.

10. **Resistance to change**: Being unwilling to adapt or pivot when faced with obstacles or setbacks can limit progress towards your goals.

** 2 **

NUTRITION ESSENTIALS: FUELING YOUR BODY FOR GROWTH

Nutrition Essentials: Fueling your body for growth likely refers to a guide or program aimed at providing essential nutrients to support physical growth and development. It would likely focus on balanced meals, proper hydration, and essential vitamins and minerals necessary for the body's growth processes. Such resources often emphasize the importance of protein for muscle development, carbohydrates for energy, healthy fats for various bodily functions, and a variety of fruits and vegetables for vitamins and minerals. It's about giving your body the right fuel to thrive and reach its full potential.

Nutrition is key for bodybuilding, supporting muscle growth, repair, and overall performance. Essential components include:

1. **Protein**: Crucial for muscle repair and growth. Aim for about 1.2-2.2 grams of protein per kilogram of body weight daily.

2. **Carbohydrates**: Provide energy for workouts and replenish glycogen stores. Choose complex carbs like whole grains, fruits, and vegetables.

3. **Fats**: Necessary for hormone production and overall health. Opt for healthy fats from sources like nuts, seeds, avocado, and fatty fish.

4. **Calories**: Consume slightly more calories than your body burns to support muscle growth, but avoid excess to prevent fat gain.

5. **Micronutrients**: Ensure adequate intake of vitamins and minerals, especially calcium, iron, vitamin D, and magnesium, which play roles in muscle function and overall health.

6. **Hydration**: Stay well-hydrated to support performance and recovery. Aim for at least 3-4 liters of water per day, adjusting based on activity level and climate.

7. **Timing**: Distribute meals and snacks evenly throughout the day to maintain energy levels and support muscle repair.

8. **Supplements**: While not essential, some supplements like protein powder, creatine, and branched-chain amino acids (BCAAs) may support muscle growth and recovery when used alongside a balanced diet.

Consistency and balance are key. Tailor your nutrition plan to your specific goals, body composition, and activity level, and consider consulting with a registered dietitian or sports nutritionist for personalized guidance.

Nutritional foods for bodybuilders typically include:

1. Lean protein sources like chicken, turkey, fish, lean beef, eggs, and plant-based proteins such as tofu, tempeh, and legumes.

2. Complex carbohydrates like sweet potatoes, brown rice, quinoa, oats, and whole grain bread.

3. Healthy fats from sources such as avocados, nuts, seeds, and olive oil.

4. Plenty of fruits and vegetables for vitamins, minerals, and antioxidants.

5. Dairy or dairy alternatives for calcium and protein, such as Greek yogurt, cottage cheese, and almond milk.

6. Hydration is crucial, so drink plenty of water throughout the day.

These foods provide essential nutrients to support muscle growth, repair, and overall performance for bodybuilders.

** 3 **

TRAINING PRINCIPLES: BODYBUILDING STRENGTH AND MUSCLE MASS

Bodybuilding revolves around principles like progressive overload, ensuring you continually challenge your muscles with heavier weights or increased resistance. Consistency is key too, maintaining a regular workout schedule and sticking to it. Proper nutrition, with a focus on protein intake for muscle repair and growth, is crucial. Adequate rest and recovery are often overlooked but essential for muscle repair and growth. And of course, form is paramount to prevent injury and maximize gains.

Here are some key training principles for bodybuilding strength and muscle mass:

1. Progressive Overload: Continuously increasing the demands on your muscles over time by lifting heavier weights or increasing resistance, which stimulates muscle growth.

2. Specificity: Tailoring your training to match your goals. For bodybuilding, this means focusing on exercises and techniques that promote hypertrophy (muscle growth) and strength.

3. Volume: The total amount of work performed in a workout, including sets, reps, and weight lifted. Increasing volume gradually can help stimulate muscle growth.

4. Intensity: Refers to how much weight you lift relative to your one-rep max (1RM). Training with high intensity, close to your 1RM, is effective for building strength and muscle mass.

5. Frequency: How often you train a muscle group or perform a particular exercise. A higher frequency can be beneficial for muscle growth, but adequate rest between sessions is crucial for recovery.

6. Rest and Recovery: Giving your muscles enough time to recover between workouts is essential for growth and preventing overtraining. This includes proper nutrition, hydration, and sleep.

7. Variation: Changing exercises, rep ranges, and training techniques to keep your muscles challenged and prevent plateaus. This can include incorporating different grips, angles, and tempos into your workouts.

8. Consistency: Regularly sticking to your training program and making gradual progress over time. Consistency is key for achieving long-term results in bodybuilding.

9. Form and Technique: Performing exercises with proper form to target the intended muscles effectively and reduce the risk of injury. Focus on controlled, deliberate movements throughout each repetition.

10. Mind-Muscle Connection: Concentrating on the muscles you're working during each exercise to maximize their activation and stimulation. This can enhance muscle growth and improve muscle control.

By incorporating these principles into your training regimen, you can optimize your workouts for building both strength and muscle mass in bodybuilding.

EXERCISES FOR BUILDING STRENGTH AND MUSCLE MASS

These are some exercises you can incorporate into your routine for building strength and muscle mass:

1. **Compound Exercises:**

- Squats
- Deadlifts
- Bench Press
- Pull-ups/Chin-ups
- Rows

2. Isolation Exercises:
- Bicep curls
- Tricep extensions
- Leg curls
- Leg extensions
- Shoulder lateral raises

3. **Core Exercises**:
- Planks
- Russian twists
- Bicycle crunches
- Hanging leg raises

4. **Functional Exercises**:
- Lunges
- Step-ups
- Push-ups
- Dips

5. **Power Exercises**:
- Power cleans
- Snatches
- Box jumps
- Medicine ball throws

Make sure to progressively increase the weights and intensity of your workouts to continue challenging your muscles and promoting growth. And don't forget to allow for adequate rest and recovery time between sessions.

** 4 **

RECOVERY STRATEGIES: MAXIMIZING STRENGTH AND REPAIR

Recovery strategies encompass a variety of techniques aimed at maximizing strength and repair after physical activity or injury. These strategies revolve around optimizing the body's natural healing processes, promoting muscle repair, and minimizing fatigue. Recovery strategies for maximizing strength and repair involve optimizing rest, nutrition, hydration, and stress management. This includes proper sleep, consuming adequate protein and nutrients, staying hydrated, and employing techniques like foam rolling, stretching, and massage to aid in muscle recovery. Additionally, incorporating active recovery exercises, such as light jogging or swimming, can promote blood flow and facilitate the removal of waste products from muscles.

To maximize strength and repair during recovery, focus on:

1. Adequate Rest: Ensure you're getting enough quality sleep to allow your body to recover and repair muscle tissue.

2. Nutrition: Consume a balanced diet with sufficient protein, carbohydrates, and healthy fats to support muscle repair and growth.

3. Hydration: Drink plenty of water to aid in the recovery process and maintain optimal performance.

4. Active Recovery: Engage in low-intensity activities like walking or stretching to promote blood flow and reduce muscle soreness.

5. Foam Rolling: Use a foam roller to massage tight muscles and improve flexibility, which can enhance recovery.

6. Proper Form: Pay attention to proper form during workouts to prevent injuries and facilitate better recovery.

7. Periodization: Incorporate planned rest days and deload weeks into your training program to prevent overtraining and promote recovery.

8. Stress Management: Manage stress through relaxation techniques such as meditation or deep breathing exercises, as excessive stress can hinder recovery.

9. Supplement Wisely: Consider supplementing with protein shakes, BCAAs, or creatine to support muscle repair and growth, but consult with a healthcare professional before starting any new supplements.

10. Listen to Your Body: Pay attention to how your body feels and adjust your training intensity and volume accordingly to prevent burnout and promote long-term progress.

FACTORS AFFECTING RECOVERY STRATEGIES

Recovery strategies can be influenced by various factors, including:

1. **Nature of the Disaster**: The type and severity of the disaster significantly impact recovery strategies. Natural disasters like earthquakes or floods may require different approaches compared to human-made disasters like cyberattacks.

2. **Resources Availability**: The availability of financial, human, and material resources greatly affects recovery strategies. Limited resources may necessitate prioritization and creative solutions.

3. **Community Resilience**: The resilience of the affected community plays a crucial role. Communities with strong social networks,

effective leadership, and disaster preparedness plans may recover more quickly.

4. **Government Policies and Support:** Government policies, funding, and support mechanisms influence the recovery process. Clear policies and efficient administration can streamline recovery efforts.

5. **Infrastructure Damage**: The extent of damage to infrastructure, including buildings, roads, utilities, and communication networks, shapes recovery strategies. Rebuilding and restoring critical infrastructure are often top priorities.

6. **Environmental Considerations:** Environmental factors such as terrain, climate, and ecological impact influence recovery strategies. Sustainable rebuilding and environmental conservation may be essential considerations.

7. **Economic Impact**: The economic consequences of the disaster, including loss of income, business disruption, and employment effects, impact recovery strategies. Economic recovery efforts often focus on restoring livelihoods and stimulating local economies.

8. **Cultural and Social Dynamics**: Cultural beliefs, social norms, and demographic characteristics shape recovery strategies. Respect for cultural practices and community engagement are essential for effective recovery.

9. **Technological Advancements**: Advances in technology, such as remote sensing, data analytics, and communication tools, can enhance recovery strategies by improving early warning systems, damage assessment, and coordination efforts.

10. **Political Stability**: Political stability and governance capacity affect recovery strategies. Political unrest or lack of effective

governance can hinder recovery efforts and exacerbate vulnerabilities.

** 5 **

ADVANCED TECHNIQUES: TAKING YOUR TRAINING TO THE NEXT LEVEL

Taking your training to the next level involves implementing advanced techniques that optimize your workouts for better results. Here are several strategies to consider:

1. **Periodization**: This involves dividing your training program into specific time periods, each with its own focus and intensity level. This can include macrocycles (annual plan), mesocycles (monthly or weekly plan), and microcycles (daily or session plan). Periodization helps prevent plateaus and overtraining by varying intensity and volume.

2. **Progressive Overload**: Continuously increasing the demands on your body over time to gradually increase strength, endurance, or muscle size. This can be achieved by increasing weight, reps, sets, or intensity of exercises.

3. **Advanced Training Techniques**:
   - **Drop Sets**: Performing a set of an exercise until failure, then immediately reducing the weight and continuing with another set.

   - **Supersets**: Performing two exercises back-to-back without rest, targeting different muscle groups.

   - **Pyramid Training**: Gradually increasing or decreasing the weight with each set while keeping the reps constant.

   - **Rest-Pause**: Pausing briefly during a set to extend the time under tension and increase intensity.

- **Negative Reps**: Emphasizing the eccentric (lowering) phase of an exercise, often with a heavier weight than you can lift concentrically (raising).

- **Isometric Holds**: Holding a position in the middle of an exercise to increase time under tension and strengthen specific joint angles.

4. **Advanced Splits**: Splitting your workouts into more targeted muscle groups or movement patterns, such as push-pull-legs, upper/lower body, or body part splits (e.g., chest and triceps one day, back and biceps another).

5. **Incorporating Functional Training**: Integrating exercises that mimic real-life movements to improve overall functional strength, stability, and mobility.

6. **Advanced Cardiovascular Training**: Implementing high-intensity interval training (HIIT), Tabata, or Fartlek training to improve cardiovascular fitness and burn more calories in a shorter amount of time.

7. **Recovery Strategies**: Prioritizing recovery with techniques such as foam rolling, stretching, yoga, massage, adequate sleep, and nutrition to optimize performance and prevent injuries.

8. **Mind-Muscle Connection**: Focusing on the contraction of the target muscle during exercises to maximize muscle recruitment and activation.

9. **Monitoring and Adjusting**: Tracking progress, listening to your body, and adjusting your training program accordingly to ensure continued progress and avoid overtraining.

10. **Advanced Nutritional Strategies**: Optimizing your nutrition for performance, including nutrient timing, macronutrient distribution, supplementation, and hydration strategies tailored to your goals and training demands.

By incorporating these advanced techniques into your training regimen, you can push past plateaus, maximize results, and take your fitness to the next level.

** 6 **

INJURY PREVENTION: SAFEGUARDING YOUR PROGRESS

Injury prevention is crucial in bodybuilding to maintain progress and avoid setbacks. Proper warm-up, stretching, and form are key. Also, ensure adequate rest between workouts and listen to your body to avoid overtraining. And don't forget to incorporate variety into your routine to prevent overuse injuries.

Injury prevention involves strategies and practices aimed at reducing the risk of injury during physical activity or exercise. It encompasses various aspects such as proper warm-up and cool-down routines, maintaining proper form and technique, using appropriate equipment, gradually increasing intensity, and listening to your body's signals. By prioritizing injury prevention, you safeguard your progress by minimizing setbacks that could hinder your fitness journey and overall well-being.

INJURY PREVENTION STRATEGIES

Here are some injury prevention strategies for bodybuilding:

1. Proper Warm-Up: Always start your workout with a dynamic warm-up to increase blood flow to the muscles and prepare them for the exercises ahead.

2. Technique Mastery: Focus on mastering proper form and technique for each exercise to reduce the risk of injury.

3. Progressive Overload: Gradually increase the intensity and load of your workouts over time to avoid overexertion and strain.

4. Rest and Recovery: Allow adequate time for rest and recovery between workouts to prevent overtraining and muscle fatigue.

5. Balanced Training: Incorporate a balanced training program that targets all major muscle groups to prevent muscular imbalances and reduce the risk of injury.

6. Listen to Your Body: Pay attention to any signs of pain or discomfort during workouts and modify exercises accordingly to prevent further injury.

7. Cross-Training: Include a variety of exercises and activities in your routine to prevent overuse injuries and keep your body balanced and resilient.

8. Proper Nutrition: Maintain a balanced diet rich in protein, carbohydrates, and healthy fats to support muscle growth and repair.

9. Hydration: Stay adequately hydrated before, during, and after workouts to support optimal muscle function and prevent cramps and fatigue.

10. Recovery Techniques: Incorporate recovery techniques such as foam rolling, stretching, and massage to alleviate muscle soreness and prevent tightness.

** 7 **

MENTAL CONDITIONING: CULTIVATING THE MINDSET OF A CHAMPION

In the realm of bodybuilding, where the difference between triumph and defeat often hinges on a razor-thin margin, the importance of mental conditioning cannot be overstated. Beyond the sweat-drenched gyms and meticulously crafted diets lies a battlefield where the mind reigns supreme. It is here, in the crucible of mental fortitude, that champions are forged.

Mental conditioning in bodybuilding transcends mere motivation or fleeting determination. It embodies a holistic approach to sculpting not just the body, but the very fabric of one's mindset. It is the unwavering belief in one's abilities, the relentless pursuit of excellence, and the resilience to overcome obstacles that defines the champion's mentality.

In this exploration of mental conditioning, we delve into the strategies, techniques, and philosophies embraced by the titans of bodybuilding. From visualization and goal setting to harnessing the power of positive affirmation, each facet contributes to the cultivation of a mindset primed for success.

But mental conditioning is not merely about pumping oneself up with superficial mantras. It is about fostering a deep-seated sense of self discipline, focus, and unwavering commitment to the journey ahead. It is about embracing the discomfort of growth and channeling it into a relentless pursuit of greatness.

Join me on a journey into the inner sanctum of the bodybuilding world, where the iron will of the mind meets the unyielding force of the body. Together, let us unlock the secrets of mental conditioning and pave the way towards achieving the mindset of a true champion in bodybuilding.

Mental conditioning in bodybuilding involves several key components:

1. Goal Setting: Setting specific, measurable, achievable, relevant, and time-bound (SMART) goals helps focus your efforts and maintain motivation.

2. Visualization: Imagining yourself achieving your goals can enhance motivation and performance by reinforcing a positive mindset.

3. Positive Self-Talk: Maintaining a positive internal dialogue can help overcome self-doubt and stay focused during challenging workouts or competitions.

4. Stress Management: Techniques such as deep breathing, meditation, and progressive muscle relaxation can help reduce stress and anxiety, enabling better focus and performance.

5. Adaptability: Being able to adapt to setbacks or unexpected challenges is crucial for maintaining resilience and staying on track towards your goals.

6. Consistency: Establishing a routine and sticking to it consistently over time is essential for progress in bodybuilding.

Cultivating these mental attributes alongside physical training can help develop the mindset of a champion in bodybuilding.

✶✶ 8 ✶✶

SUPPLEMENT GUIDE: ENHANCING PERFORMANCE SAFELY

In the world of bodybuilding, achieving peak performance and maximizing gains is a continuous pursuit. While proper nutrition, training, and rest are fundamental pillars, many athletes turn to supplements to enhance their results further. However, the realm of supplements can be complex and overwhelming, with a plethora of options promising various benefits.

This guide aims to provide clarity and guidance on safely incorporating supplements into your bodybuilding regimen to optimize performance and promote overall well-being. From protein powders to pre-workouts and beyond, understanding the science behind each supplement, its potential benefits, and the safest practices for consumption is crucial for achieving sustainable progress.

We'll delve into evidence-based recommendations, highlighting the supplements with the most substantial research backing and those that align with your specific fitness goals. Additionally, we'll discuss key considerations such as dosage, timing, and potential side effects to ensure that you approach supplementation with informed decision-making and prioritize safety above all else.

Whether you're a seasoned bodybuilder looking to fine-tune your routine or a newcomer eager to maximize your results, this supplement guide will serve as a comprehensive resource to help you navigate the vast landscape of bodybuilding supplements effectively and safely.

Here's a guide to supplements commonly used in bodybuilding, along with explanations of how they can enhance performance safely:

1. Protein Powder: Essential for muscle repair and growth, especially post-workout. Look for whey, casein, or plant-based options.

2. Creatine: Improves strength and power output by increasing ATP production in muscles. It's one of the most researched supplements and considered safe.

3. BCAAs (Branched-Chain Amino Acids): Leucine, isoleucine, and valine aid in muscle recovery, reduce muscle soreness, and promote muscle growth.

4. Beta-Alanine: Increases muscle endurance by buffering lactic acid buildup, allowing for longer and more intense workouts.

5. Caffeine: Enhances energy, focus, and endurance, making it beneficial for intense training sessions. It's safe in moderate doses but can cause side effects in excessive amounts.

6. Fish Oil: Rich in omega-3 fatty acids, it reduces inflammation, supports heart health, and may improve muscle recovery.

7. Multivitamin: Ensures adequate micronutrient intake, which is crucial for overall health and optimal performance.

8. Vitamin D: Supports bone health, immune function, and muscle strength. Many people have deficient levels, especially those with limited sun exposure.

9. Glutamine: Helps with muscle recovery and immune system function, particularly during periods of intense training or calorie restriction.

10. ZMA (Zinc, Magnesium, Vitamin B6): Supports testosterone production, muscle recovery, and quality sleep, all of which are important for performance and muscle growth.

Always consult with a healthcare professional before starting any new supplement regimen, especially if you have any pre-existing medical conditions or are taking medication.

Additionally, remember that supplements are meant to complement a balanced diet and consistent training routine, not replace them.

✳✳ 9 ✳✳

CASE STUDIES: REAL-LIFE EXAMPLES OF SUCCESSFUL BODYBUILDERS

Bodybuilding is not just about lifting weights; it's a lifestyle that requires dedication, discipline, and persistence. While the gym is where the muscles are built, the journey to success often involves more than just physical strength.

Case studies offer invaluable insights into the real-life experiences of successful bodybuilders, shedding light on their training routines, diet plans, mindset, and the challenges they faced along the way. By examining these case studies, aspiring bodybuilders can learn from the triumphs and setbacks of those who have already achieved success in the sport.

In this introduction, we'll explore how case studies provide a window into the world of bodybuilding, offering practical lessons and inspiration for anyone looking to improve their physique and performance. Through the stories of accomplished bodybuilders, we'll uncover the strategies and principles that have helped them reach the pinnacle of their sport, demonstrating that with the right mindset and approach, anyone can achieve their fitness goals.

Here are a few real-life examples of successful bodybuilders:

1. Arnold Schwarzenegger: Perhaps the most iconic bodybuilder of all time, Arnold won Mr. Olympia seven times and went on to become a successful actor and politician.

2. Ronnie Coleman: A legendary figure in bodybuilding, Coleman holds the record for most Mr. Olympia wins, with eight victories.

3. Jay Cutler: A four-time Mr. Olympia winner, Cutler is known for his incredible size and symmetry on the bodybuilding stage.

4. Dorian Yates: Yates dominated bodybuilding in the 1990s, winning the Mr. Olympia title six times with his intense training style and focus on muscle mass.

5. Lee Haney: Haney won the Mr. Olympia title eight times, tying with Ronnie Coleman for the second-most wins in the history of the competition.

These bodybuilders achieved success through a combination of dedicated training, strict dieting, and unwavering discipline, inspiring countless others in the fitness community.

** 10 **

CONCLUSION: SUSTAINING LONG-TERM SUCCESS IN BODYBUILDING

To sustain long-term success in bodybuilding, it's essential to prioritize consistency in training, nutrition, and recovery. This means following a well-rounded workout program, maintaining a balanced diet rich in nutrients, and allowing adequate time for rest and recovery to prevent burnout and injury. Additionally, setting realistic goals, staying committed, and continually educating oneself on effective training methods and nutrition strategies are crucial for long-term progress in bodybuilding.

Sustaining long-term success in bodybuilding requires a multifaceted approach:

1. Consistent Training: Stick to a well-designed workout plan that includes resistance training and progressive overload to continuously challenge your muscles.

2. Proper Nutrition: Fuel your body with a balanced diet rich in protein, complex carbohydrates, healthy fats, vitamins, and minerals to support muscle growth and recovery.

3. Adequate Rest and Recovery: Allow your muscles to recover by getting enough sleep and incorporating rest days into your training schedule. Overtraining can lead to burnout and injury.

4. Monitoring Progress: Track your progress by keeping a workout journal, taking regular measurements, and assessing your strength and physique improvements over time.

About

A.B.O. Comix is a collective of creators and activists who work to amplify the voices of LGBTQ prisoners through art. By working closely with prison abolitionist and queer advocacy organizations, we aim to keep queer prisoners connected to outside community and help them in the fight toward liberation. The profits we generate go back to incarcerated artists, especially those with little to no resources. Using the DIY ideology of "punk-zine" culture, A.B.O. Comix was formed with the philosophy of mutual support, community, and friendship.

Our collective is working towards compassionate accountability without relying on the state or its sycophants. A.B.O. Comix believes our interpersonal and societal issues can be solved without locking people in cages. Our mission is to combat the culture that treats humans as disposable and disproportionately criminalizes the most marginalized amongst us. Through artistic activism, we hope to proliferate the idea that a better world means redefining our concepts of justice.

Find us online at www.abocomix.com

With love and solidarity,
A.B.O. Comix Collective

5. Adjustment and Adaptation: Be willing to adjust your training and nutrition based on your progress, goals, and any plateaus you encounter. This might involve changing exercises, increasing weights, or modifying your diet.

6. Mindset and Motivation: Develop a positive mindset and stay motivated by setting realistic goals, celebrating achievements, and finding inspiration from within or through mentors and peers.

7. Injury Prevention: Prioritize proper form during exercises, warm up adequately before workouts, and listen to your body to avoid injuries that could derail your progress.

8. Lifestyle Factors: Manage stress levels, avoid excessive alcohol and drug use, and prioritize overall health to support your bodybuilding endeavors in the long run.

By consistently implementing these strategies, you can sustain long-term success in bodybuilding while minimizing setbacks and maximizing progress.